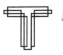

The little book of
BIG
WEIGHT LOSS™

Bernadette Fisers

TOUCHSTONE

New York   London   Toronto   Sydney   New Delhi

Touchstone
An Imprint of Simon & Schuster, Inc.
1230 Avenue of the Americas
New York, NY 10020

First Touchstone trade paperback edition December 2017

TOUCHSTONE and colophon are registered trademarks of Simon & Schuster, Inc.

For information about special discounts for bulk purchases, please contact Simon & Schuster Special Sales at 1-866-506-1949 or business@simonandschuster.com.

The Simon & Schuster Speakers Bureau can bring authors to your live event. For more information or to book an event, contact the Simon & Schuster Speakers Bureau at 1-866-248-3049 or visit our website at www.simonspeakers.com.

Interior design by Myrtle Jeffs
Vector drawings by Leremy/Shutterstock

Manufactured in the United States of America

10   9   8   7   6   5   4   3   2   1

Library of Congress Cataloging-in-Publication Data
Names: Fisers, Bernadette, author.
Title: The little book of big weight loss / Bernadette Fisers.
Description: First Touchstone trade paperback edition. | New York : Touchstone, 2018. | Originally published in Australia in 2016. | Includes bibliographical references.
Identifiers: LCCN 2017043005| ISBN 9781501183782 (paperback) | ISBN 9781501183799 (ebook)
Subjects: LCSH: Weight loss—Popular works. | Reducing diets—Popular works. | BISAC: HEALTH & FITNESS / Weight Loss. | HEALTH & FITNESS / Nutrition. | COOKING / Health & Healing / Weight Control.
Classification: LCC RM222.2 .F49 2018 | DDC 613.2/5—dc23 LC record available at https://lccn.loc.gov/2017043005

ISBN 978-1-5011-8378-2
ISBN 978-1-5011-8379-9 (ebook)

for my daughter, Lilli,
may she never have the weight problems i've had

contents

hello :)

. . . welcome to a healthier and slimmer you . . .

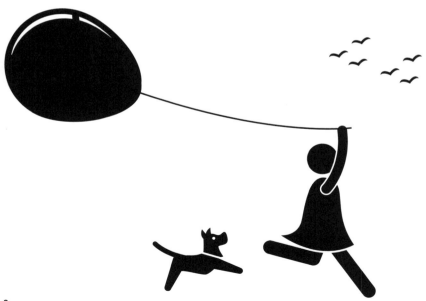

it's not fun being fat—or, to be politically correct, overweight. i should know. once upon a time, i was seriously overweight too—in fact, i was massive.

I'm a full-time working mom. Like many in the same situation, I was time poor and didn't make myself a priority. At my worst, I weighed over a staggering (and uncomfortable) 283 pounds. At 5'7" tall, that made my BMI a huge 41.8 percent. In medical speak? I was morbidly obese.

To change things, I desperately needed to know what to do in order to drop weight and be healthy—fast. I was fat and getting fatter by the minute, as well as on the brink of diabetes, with hypertension (high blood pressure) and a fatty liver. My doctor was freaking out—and I don't blame her.

I had read enough of the boring and expensive diet books that were 300 pages long but had only a couple of useful points in them. I didn't need some superfit trainer speculating on how to lose weight from their lofty six-pack perch—I wanted someone who *truly understood* the physical and emotional toll, someone who had lived through their own weight issues and who had also been through successful weight loss—someone who could get to the point simply and quickly. And I didn't want some of the answers—I needed all of them!

the bad news: obesity is a global health epidemic.

the good news: there is a simple solution for many.

The US surgeon general states that obesity increases the risk of developing cardiovascular disease, type 2 diabetes, hypertension and some cancers. The cost to the United States is estimated to range from $147 billion to nearly $210 billion per year. Isn't that terrifying? I'm sure those billions could be used better elsewhere. According to the World Health Organization (WHO) the United States has one of the highest incidences of obesity in the English-speaking world, with a whopping 74.1 percent of the population either overweight or obese. The United Kingdom and Australia have very similar obesity figures.

We have always been told to eat less and exercise more; for years, that has been the commonsense answer to losing weight. But . . . well . . . *what if that's wrong?* We've also been told that it's our fault we are fat—we're "too lazy, too greedy," or we don't have the willpower, plus a barrage of other insulting stuff.

That is also a *big fat lie.*

Why are more of us obese than ever before? It's obvious: we've been given the wrong advice.

so stop putting yourself down and read this— i mean read it and absorb it— because this works . . . *fast*

Supermarkets are a minefield of sugary food and drinks—and unfortunately, the average shopper is misled again and again. How are you supposed to know what's truly healthful when every second food product is labeled "diet" or "lite," but will actually make you fatter?

There are many false beliefs about what's going to help. My method of weight loss costs nothing; it's simply a shift in how you shop and eat. In doing so, I lost 66 pounds in thirty weeks.

I know! WTF? Pause while I high-five myself!

I was uncomfortable. I was fat. I was desperate for a long-term answer—and nothing was working. So I started reading and doing research, looking at recent medical studies on losing weight and asking the people I work with—mostly young, fit models—what they eat.

I became my own guinea pig. When one weight loss technique worked, I found ways to boost it. *I wanted to achieve the fastest weight loss possible without killing myself doing it.* A way of dropping the weight that would last over the long haul, as I had a lot of weight to lose.

I wanted warp-speed weight loss. When you're fat, you want the fat gone—preferably yesterday. *I wanted the fat to stay off— permanently.* This weight loss plan had to be something I could commit to for life. A lifestyle change for the better.

Individually, the techniques in this book are not new. But put together, just like combining hydrogen and oxygen to make water (H_2O), they're like magic. It's this *combination of techniques* that creates superfast weight loss. And, as a by-product, improved health. (Obviously, get yourself checked out by your doctor too.)

I know you have a busy life, so this book is a condensed, quick read—simple ideas that work. Big weight loss is *mostly about the food.* Exercise is important to a lesser extent—for me, it's walking and, in summer, swimming. This year in a bikini . . .

I follow these rules every day.

while everyone is different, here are the health benefits i gained from eating like this . . .

- weight loss (66 pounds . . . so far)
- stable blood sugar
- lower risk of diabetes
- better blood pressure
- lower cholesterol
- less visceral fat (the bad fat around organs)
- less inflammation in my body
- improved liver function
- more energy
- less fatigue
- great mood
- glowing skin
- sharper brain
- better clothes to buy! (and i'm not invisible to salepeople)
- easier to run around with kids
- positive life outlook
- pride in myself
- better concentration
- people say i look 10 years younger
- looking forward to exercising
- feeling AMAZING

"great things are done not by impulse but by a series of small things brought together."

—vincent van gogh

here are the rules that i live by every day . . .

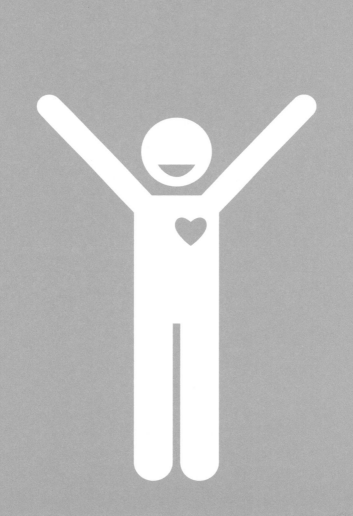

rules for the body

these rules all contributed to giving me the fastest weight loss possible; together they are magic.

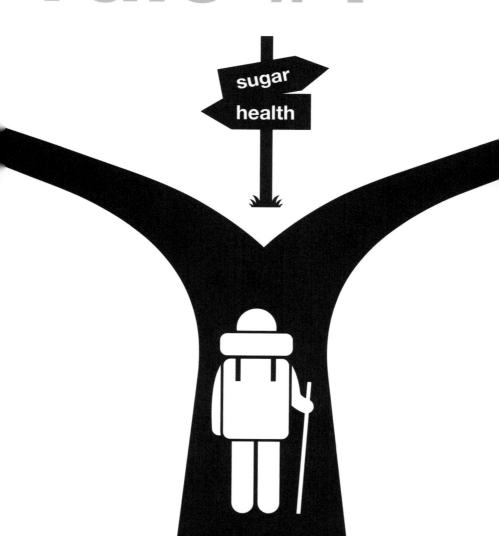

. . . i don't eat sugar, especially fructose . . .

why?

it makes you fat and it's addictive. it's that simple.

there are dozens of names for sugar, no wonder we don't even know when we're eating it.

Agave nectar, Barbados sugar, barley malt, barley malt syrup, beet sugar, brown sugar, cane juice, cane juice crystals, cane sugar, caramel, carob syrup, caster sugar, coconut palm sugar, coconut sugar, confectioner's sugar, corn sweetener, corn syrup, corn syrup solids, date sugar, dehydrated cane juice, demerara sugar, dextrin, dextrose, evaporated cane juice, pourable brown sugar, fructose, fruit juice, fruit juice concentrate, glucose, glucose solids, golden syrup, grape sugar, HFCS (high-fructose corn syrup), honey, icing sugar, invert sugar, malt syrup, maltodextrin, maltose, mannose, maple syrup, molasses, muscovado sugar, palm sugar, panocha, powdered sugar, raw sugar, refiner's syrup, rice syrup, saccharose, sorghum syrup, sucrose, sugar (granulated), sweet sorghum, syrup, turbinado sugar

Fructose is in everything. Who knew? It was a major factor in my being overweight, as I have a real sweet tooth.

Chocolate cookies would positively call my name. I could demolish a pack of Mallomars in ten minutes flat. That's 100.8 grams of sugar, or over 25 teaspoons.

Sugar is not just in sweets, though. It can also be found in many savory foods, such as BBQ sauce, which can be up to 50 percent sugar. Isn't that an astounding fact?

Food companies call it "the bliss point": adding sugar to sweet *and* savory foods to make them more palatable—and more addictive.

Added sugars are found in approximately 75 percent of food at the supermarket, including in things that you wouldn't expect, such as bread. The highest concentration of sugars is found mostly in these foods: sweetened beverages, baked goods, dairy desserts, candy and—wait for it— breakfast cereals. Isn't that horrifying?

I aim to stick to fewer than 3 added teaspoons of sugar a day. A teaspoon is 4 grams. In general, the less sugar in my diet, the faster my weight loss. This is my most important rule; I equate it to 50 percent of my weight loss.

this is how sugar can make you fat.

In general, eating too much sugar will make you fat, but there is something else to remember: all sugars are not equal. There are two common forms of sugar, fructose and glucose. White sugar is a combination of the two. Fructose, when overconsumed, does not send a message to the brain to stop eating; glucose does. Unfortunately, fructose is found in most of our sweet foods and some of our savory foods.

In other words, you are fat and not full, so you keep eating. The more you eat, the more you want—it's a vicious cycle. Think about how easy it is to eat a heap of sweet food and never feel full. Usually I get to the "feel sick" stage first.

Sugar turns into fat right away—unless you're an Olympic athlete or superactive and burn it—and has a toxic effect on your body when overconsumed.

It's also seriously addictive (as you may have noticed)—even more than cocaine, as proven by several reliable medical studies.

You will need to be strong and consistently say no to break this sugar addiction, but once you do, it's an amazing difference.

It doesn't take long to get off sugar; it takes determination. Within a week or so you should be feeling great: less tired, with more energy, fewer bad moods and a more positive outlook, among other benefits.

I am no longer addicted. I no longer feel the desire to reach out and throw three bars of chocolate in my cart when shopping, then eat one on the way home. I didn't realize how addicted I was, but now it's easy to say **no**.

rule #2

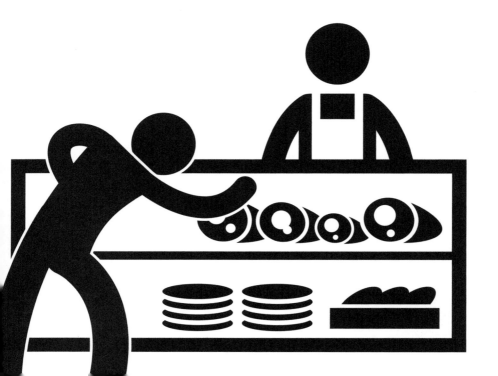

. . . i mostly don't eat processed foods . . .

unfortunately, about 80 percent of the supermarket is made up of processed foods.

such as:
potato chips
cookies
chocolate bars
sauces
breakfast cereals
(most are high in
sugar)
salad dressings
canned fruit
frozen French
fries

and that's only a
small sample!

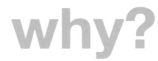

why?

There are heaps of processed foods in the supermarket (about 80 percent), which means lots of hidden added sugars, bad fats and added salt—and all these foods can make you fat. *Yes, even savory food.*

Since the 1960s, food has been more and more processed. Think about it: before the 1960s, there wasn't much of a problem with obesity. *In fact, obesity rates have more than tripled since then.*

There also weren't many processed foods. People mostly cooked at home and ate relatively simply. Now it's hard to go out shopping anywhere without finding food by the checkout counter.

When prepackaged and processed foods were first introduced, some companies put extra sugar into their products. Sugar is cheap and addictive, making you want to eat more and therefore buy more—it's called "the bliss point." *Smart for business but bad for your health.*

When you eat supposed "healthful" processed foods, you can end up consuming lots of hidden sugars, not to mention lots of synthetic chemicals, which is far from natural.

For example, a small (13-ounce) can of baked beans has the equivalent of an added 5 teaspoons of sugar in it. (A teaspoon is 4 grams.)

Ketchup is full of sugar—high-fructose corn syrup, to be precise. Plus other ingredients that I don't recognize. Considering that 1 tablespoon of a popular ketchup contains 1 teaspoon of sugar, it is very easy to load 3 teaspoons of sugar onto a burger. Imagine actually scooping those 3 teaspoons onto your food—that is effectively what you are doing. Surprising, isn't it?

The US National Health and Nutrition Examination Survey 2009–2010 says, "Decreasing the consumption of ultraprocessed foods could be an effective way of reducing the excessive intake of added sugars in the USA." No kidding!

rule #3

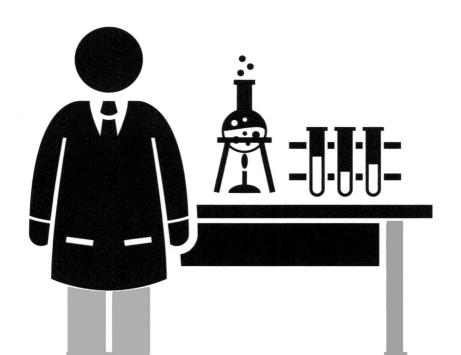

. . . i don't drink fizzy drinks (soda) or fruit juices, ever . . .

such as:
canned or bottled
soda, iced teas
and coffees or fruit
juices in any form.

this is a really
important rule for
those who love
sweet drinks.

why?

sodas, iced teas, juices and some coffees are full of sugar and can make you fat. don't drink your way to fatness— it's easily done.

As an experiment, try to eat the equivalent amount of fruit that makes up a juice— say, five or six apples. You can't. The fruit makes you full; that's the fiber filling you up.

If we were meant to juice our fruits, I'm pretty sure they would have come with a straw attached—clearly they don't.

Sodas contain between 10 and 12 teaspoons of sugar per 12-ounce can, depending on which you choose. Iced teas can contain up to 12 teaspoons per 16-ounce bottle, and a Frappuccino contains about 10 teaspoons of sugar. Considering that I want to consume only about 3 added teaspoons of sugar a day, all these are definitely off the menu.

The sugar-free diet ones are full of chemicals such as phosphoric acid, aspartame, potassium benzonate . . . I don't even know what they are, let alone want to drink them.

Some people believe that there is nothing wrong with drinking a diet soda that contains zero calories. It's really up to you whether or not you are happy to consume the chemicals. For me, it is a no.

So I don't drink any of them. Except seltzer.

Juices are full of fructose (sugar), without the benefit of the fiber that has been removed (the fiber is the good bit). A typical glass of apple juice has 7.5 teaspoons of sugar, which is a lot!

In short, juices have all of the sugar content (bad stuff) but none of the fiber content (good stuff). The fiber keeps your blood sugar stable and helps you feel much fuller. If your fruit is organic, try not to peel it; the peel contains a lot of fiber.

Which leads to the next rule . . .

rule #4

. . . i drink plenty of water . . .

why?

I drink about six to eight glasses of water a day. More in summer.

Water is essential to life. And it's essential to feeling good and dropping weight. I drink still or sparkling water, and I try to aim for eight glasses a day. I find this easier to do in summer than winter. **If you feel thirsty, it means you're already dehydrated**. So drink up.

I do not drink flavored waters. I do, occasionally, put some fresh lemon into my water. Try to drink water 15 minutes before eating. It makes you feel fuller and therefore eat less. I put a glass of water next to my plate at every meal to encourage me to drink it.

Drink water first thing in the morning. It sets you up for the day. Remember, water is your calorie-free friend.

Sometimes when I'm stalking the fridge and hunting around for something, it's actually water that I want—not food. It's surprisingly easy to get mixed up about what you actually need. Sounds weird, but it's true for me.

organic apple cider vinegar
(buy one containing mother).

When I remember, I take 2 teaspoons of apple cider vinegar in a glass of water. This helps to increase good gut bacteria. I do this up to twice a day. Dilute the vingar with water; otherwise it will ruin your teeth!

rule #5

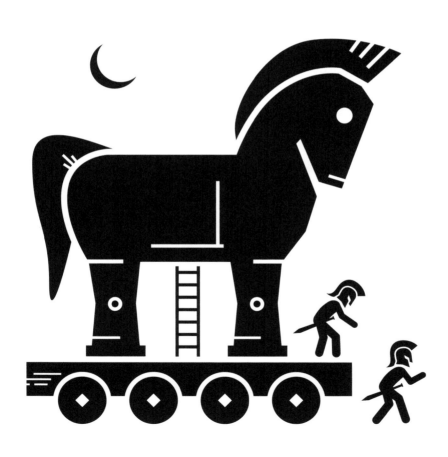

. . . i don't buy diet or low-fat foods . . .

such as:
diet or lite yogurt
low-fat yogurt
skim milk
low-fat milk
diet cookies
diet desserts
diet dressings

i eat:
full-fat greek yogurt
full-fat cheese
full-fat milk
cream
sour cream
butter

why?

diet or lite foods are usually full of sugar and salt to compensate for the lack of taste from missing fats, and they *will make you fatter*—not thinner, as their name implies.

Let's take diet yogurt. It should really be called pudgy yogurt—but I doubt that would sell. And as we know, it's all about what sells—unfortunately at our expense.

A popular diet yogurt—a small tub, 150 grams, about 1 cup of yogurt, the size you would give a kid to take to school—contains 36 grams or 9 teaspoons of sugar. The way the food companies try to fool you is by saying that the small tub has 4 servings in it. Yeah, right! Like I would eat 2 spoonfuls and then put it back into the fridge. Hello! I mean, seriously . . . in total, that's more sugar than in a candy bar!

I try to eat as little added sugar as possible, so this is not even an option. No pudgy yogurt! I usually buy full-fat Greek yogurt or coconut yogurt with a very low sugar content.

The same rule goes for milk, cheese—all dairy products. I buy the full-fat version of everything. Full-fat dairy products make you feel fuller for longer. Natural fats fill you up and eliminate the hungry feeling.

Dairy products are a good source of calcium, protein, iodine, vitamin A, vitamin D, riboflavin, vitamin B_{12} and zinc.

Obviously, don't go crazy on dairy products! And check the sugar and salt content. I probably consume 1 cup of milk, plus 1 ounce (30g) of cheese a day; perhaps some sour cream and/or butter in my cooking.

There is speculation that cutting back on dairy products is good for some people; this isn't the case for me, as I am not lactose intolerant.

rule #6

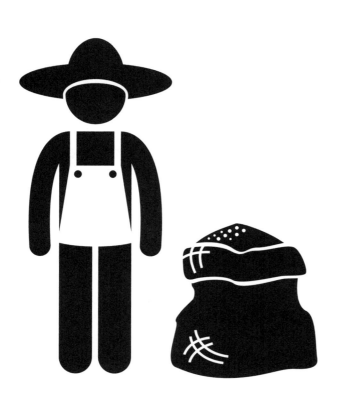

. . . i seriously cut back on carbs—processed and refined— *and i mean seriously* . . .

why?

i do not eat white bread, pasta or white potatoes.

Breads, pastas and potatoes are all carbs that I used to love eating to excess. Athletes may need them for energy, but I am no professional athlete, and I don't need that kind of energy for what I do day to day.

Essentially, I'm now eating lower carb. I'm certainly not saying no carb—vegetables are carbs, too!

I'm saying: lower calorie, more nutritious carbs.

In general, I swap white bread, pasta and potatoes to higher-fiber, more nutritious food such as vegetables, which are generally lower in calories. I want my body to use its many stored fats instead.

If you're desperate for pasta, pick up a spiralizer, which turns veggies such as zucchini into something resembling pasta but much healthier. It is fun to use—my daughter loves it.

Bread can be tricky. I don't know about you, but I have a love affair with bread. You need to buy a whole grain bread plus check the label, as many have hidden sugars—or, better still, bake your own (see Bern's Simple High-Protein Bread Recipe on the facing page). I know, it sounds tedious—but it's actually really quick. A home-baked loaf takes me about ten minutes to make and lasts me a week.

I bake with lentil or chickpea flour, which are both higher in protein and fiber and have about one-quarter the carb content of regular white flour. And they're gluten free—if you're into that. I eat two slices of my protein bread a day and it's seriously yummy and filling.

Put simply, your body requires more energy to burn protein (fish, meat, eggs, etc.). About double, in fact. It's called the thermic effect. So think lean protein and natural fats, with a large healthy dose of vegetables and water. This will make you feel fuller longer.

Eating this way will make you less sluggish, as your blood sugars will be more balanced. I now have fewer peaks and crashes throughout the day. I also don't feel bloated at all, and I find that I have more energy for longer!

bread

Swap to a bread made with chickpea, quinoa or lentil flour—it is significantly lower in carbohydrates than white flour, but higher in protein, iron and fiber and will make you feel fuller longer. Better still, bake your own. I eat no more than two slices a day. At the very least buy a whole grain, low-sugar bread.

potatoes

Swap white potatoes to sweet potatoes, which have a higher vitamin content. I would eat sweet potato only once a week—and only about a quarter of one.

rice

Brown and wild rice is higher in fiber than white rice. I would have no more than a half cup of rice (cooked) per week. Swap to quinoa or chia, as they are higher in protein.

pasta

No pasta—I tend to eat it to excess, unfortunately.

It's all about the quality of the carbohydrates that you are eating.

bern's simple high-protein bread recipe (gf)

2 eggs
1 teaspoon salt
1 zucchini, grated
1 large carrot, grated
1 teaspoon baking soda
2 cups chickpea flour
½ cup organic coconut oil, melted
1 teaspoon turmeric
2 tablespoons dukkah (Egyptian spice blend)
If the mixture feels a bit dry, add some yogurt or hummus—a couple of tablespoons.

Preheat convection oven to 350°F degrees, fan forced. Mix all the ingredients together until just combined, and pour into a loaf tin. Bake for about 50 minutes.

When done, it should be medium brown and probably cracked on top; when you insert a skewer, it should come out clean. You can substitute other herbs and spices for different versions—I've put in oregano, garlic, basil. Plus I often add sunflower seeds.

I store it in the refrigerator, it lasts me a week and I eat it toasted. Enjoy!

rule #7

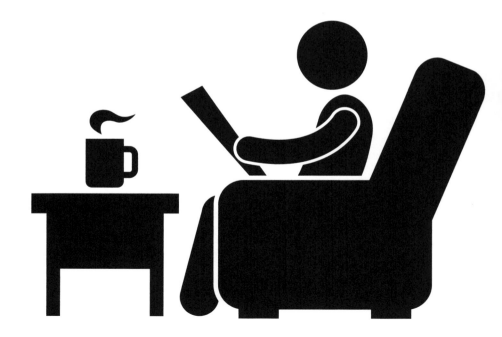

. . . i finish eating at 7 p.m. and don't eat again until 10 a.m. . . .

when fasting at night, your body goes into repair mode, correcting blood sugar levels and burning stored fats. who knew? it's amazing.

it's called
intermittent fasting,
and it works. it's
not a diet, it's a
pattern of eating.

the maximum
time for a woman
to fast overnight is
fourteen to fifteen
hours—for men it
is sixteen.

i fast for fifteen,
and it works great
for me.

why?

We live in an eating society. We're always eating, and we don't tend to give ourselves a break from it. But we should; our bodies need it.

Overnight is an easy time to do an intermittent fast. Fasting lowers insulin levels, increases growth hormone levels and increases the amount of a brain chemical called norepinephrine, all of which encourage the breakdown of body fat and facilitate its use for energy.

For this reason, short-term fasting actually increases your metabolic rate by up to 14 percent, helping you burn even more calories. Fasting is an excellent way to reboot your system.

It's not hard to do; you're mostly sleeping anyway. I do this every night, except when my social life collides with it. That's when I cut myself some slack and start again the next day.

You may think that you'll wake up ravenous and run screaming to the fridge—but in fact that doesn't happen. It's almost the opposite. Weird, hey?

How I do it: breakfast after 10 a.m., lunch around 2 p.m. and dinner around 6 p.m. Because there are fewer hours between meals, I tend to eat less in between. On a hungry day I might snack on nuts, cheese or veggies.

During my fasting period—7 p.m. to 10 a.m.—I drink green tea at night and strong coffee in the morning.

I find giving my body this rest period extremely beneficial, as I feel so much better for it. I don't see myself stopping it in either the short or long term. I love it.

rule #8

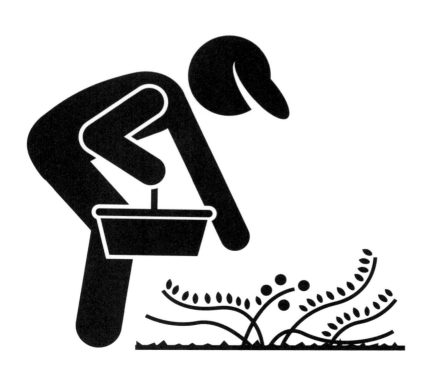

. . . i limit my fruit to 1 or 2 pieces a day. i eat the whole fruit—don't juice it . . .

berries are always
my first choice.

also, i do not eat
dried fruits.

why?

don't juice it or peel it, as you will lose the fiber, which is the good bit.

Fruit contains fructose—but not all fruits are equal. For example, berries, grapefruit and nectarines have less fructose (sugar) than a mango or watermelon. Choose well—but don't beat yourself up about it. Grapes are high in fructose, so I tend to stay away from those.

If organic, eat the whole fruit, including the skin if possible. Don't juice it; otherwise you're losing all the good bits, namely the fiber, which helps you lose weight and aids in digestion. I limit the amount of fruit I eat because I want the fastest possible weight loss and fruit contains a lot of fructose/sugar—**and I am on a mission.**

Sometimes I will have only one serving a day, usually berries, which are lower in fructose and high in fiber. Though perhaps I'm scarred from when I was a kid and would come home from school and say, "I'm starved." My mom would always say, "Have a piece of fruit." Aaaaahhh!

Eat fruits when they're in season; they are generally fresher. A farmers' market is a good place to buy fresh fruit and veggies—really fresh and natural.

Dried fruits are generally high in fructose/ sugar. You might as well be popping candy into your mouth. A half-cup serving of dates contains about 55 grams of fructose, which is the equivalent of 14 teaspoons of sugar. Regardless of where it comes from, your body treats sugar the same way—by turning it into fat—so I avoid dried fruits.

rule #9

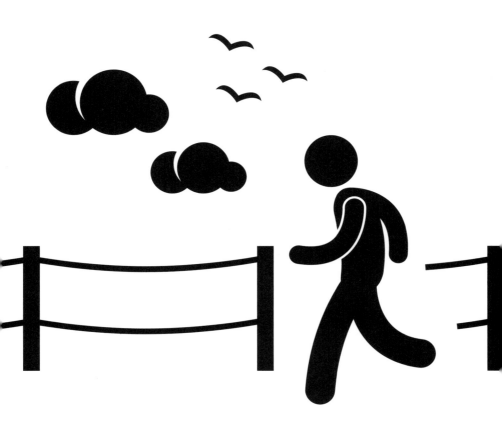

. . . i walk at least 10,000 steps a day or exercise for the equivalent . . .

wear a pedometer or download a walking app; it's easier than you think, and i think of it as my time. i go for a walk and listen to music or a podcast. i also come back in a better mood.

this is an important rule: exercise is great for my mental well-being, and feeling good helps me stay on track.

Taking 10,000 steps a day is a rough equivalent of the guideline to do 150 minutes of activity a week—i.e., 25 minutes every day. According to the US surgeon general, "Physical activity strengthens bones and muscles, reduces stress and depression and makes it easier to maintain a healthy body weight or to reduce weight if overweight or obese." It's enough exercise to reduce your risk of disease and help you lead a longer, healthier life. The benefits are many: lower BMI, reduced waist size, increased energy and less risk of developing type 2 diabetes and heart disease.

On average, a regular 2-ounce chocolate bar is 270 calories—to burn that off, you'd have to walk for an hour. If you want to actually lose weight but not change your eating habits, you'll need to exercise full-time, and none of us has time for that!

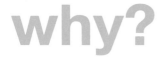

why?

exercise burns fat, makes you feel fabulous and helps with general well-being. it also increases your muscle mass, which helps burn fat faster.

I don't know about you, but I absolutely do not have time to turn into a gym bunny.

Samuel Klein, MD, at the Washington University School of Medicine, says, "Decreasing food intake is much more effective than increasing physical activity to achieve weight loss." No kidding!

Luckily for me and, hopefully, you, serious weight loss is mostly about the food—combined with a reasonable amount of exercise. Ditch the Lycra, get out your pedometer and start walking.

When you do get the desire to do more—and you will, believe it or not!—I suggest lifting weights as well as doing cardio such as walking, running, etc. Weight training builds muscle—which not only makes you look more toned and slimmer but also burns fat. Win-win!

And yes, exercise does make you hungrier, so don't pig out after it. Have a healthful snack and plenty of water instead. You'll feel doubly as good!

Exercise alone will never be enough to lose a significant amount of weight, because you have to do a TON in order to burn large amounts of fat. **That's why what you put in your mouth is so important.**

rule #10

. . . i always read food labels . . .

why?

you need to know the ingredients in what you are buying and eating.

knowledge will speed up your weight loss.

let's face it, food labels are confusing. however, there's an easy rule! the shorter the label, the better. when there are lots of ingredients, it usually means more processing.

For example, canned chickpeas. The ingredient list: chickpeas and water. Great!

Generally, the fewer ingredients, the better. Stay away from anything with trans fats, as well as significant added sugar and salt. Remember, 4 grams is a teaspoon.

When I first started reading labels, if I saw an ingredient I didn't recognize, I wouldn't buy it. As a rule, ingredients are listed by order of volume—i.e., the first ingredient listed comprises the majority of the product.

Think about this: you don't need a food label on an apple. The best food for you is a whole ingredient. Really, anything that requires a food label—or is advertised on TV—is a bit suspect, and the smaller the number of ingredients the better. But in reality, we're all busy, and sometimes convenience wins out.

Just be smart about what you throw into your cart and what you feed your family—especially your kids. Teach them how to eat properly. It will save them from having the weight issues that you have had.

I ask my daughter to run on ahead of me and find the can of tomatoes with the lowest amount of sugar. It's great—she's learning, plus saving me time. Win-win.

Doing this will quickly become a habit. You know those lean and healthy people standing in the supermarket studying labels? That will soon be you!

rule #11

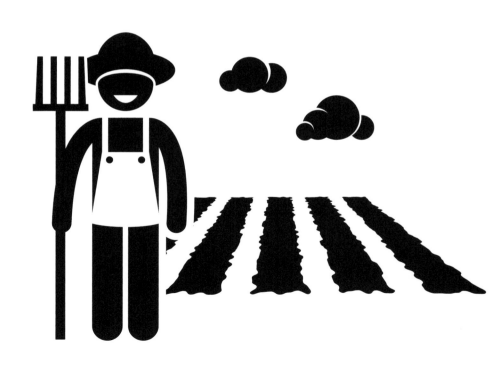

. . . i eat whole foods . . .

such as: eggs, vegetables, fish, meat, fruit (the whole fruit), grains, beans, dairy, nuts.

whole foods are single-ingredient foods, usually with no ingredient list. they can be combined with other single ingredients to make delicious meals.

why?

it's back to simplicity.
shop simply.

You know exactly what you're getting—there are no hidden sugars or fats or synthetic chemicals.

There is a *reason* why most slim celebrities I work with have specific dietary requirements—it's because *they are all eating whole foods*, not because they are being difficult.

I also try to eat fruit and veggies only when they're in season—why eat six-month-old canned fruit or something that's been stored or treated with gas to preserve it?

When I was working on an ad for a supermarket chain, I went out to a storage dungeon for apples, and it wasn't pretty—more like pretty gross. Stick to fresh and organic if you can.

I prefer organic chicken, grass-fed beef, free-range pork. Buy meats and fish produced where the animals are treated as humanely as possible. I limit my red meat consumption to once a week, mostly due to the health benefits of eating it sparingly. I always choose fish or chicken first. Processed meats are an absolute no-no. The high consumption of red and processed meats has been linked with some cancers, according to the World Health Organization.

Adding spices and seasoning to your food boosts flavor and taste, which will help you feel satisfied. In winter, I use my slow cooker, and in summer, I make lots of salads—simple!

rule #12

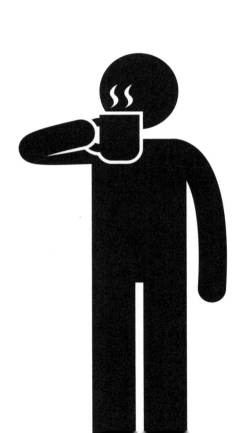

. . . i drink coffee first thing . . .

why?

i do this first thing in the morning when i wake up, then wait to have my breakfast at 10 a.m.

The caffeine kick-starts my metabolism. It's a tip from some of the celebrity fitness gurus and athletes I've worked with. They all say the same thing about the morning coffee—plus it helps keep me regular—bonus!

The caffeine in coffee increases the rate at which your body burns calories. I stick to two cups per day. I drink mine with a touch of milk (it's called a piccolo latte)—full fat, of course. The reason I want only a touch of milk is that it is lower in calories than, say, a full caffe latte, which contains a full cup of milk and, therefore, triple the calories. Sometimes I will use coconut milk in my coffee, as I like the taste and it has fewer calories than full-fat milk.

If you have issues with caffeine such as headaches or jitters, avoid it and drink caffeine-free green tea or water instead.

rule #13

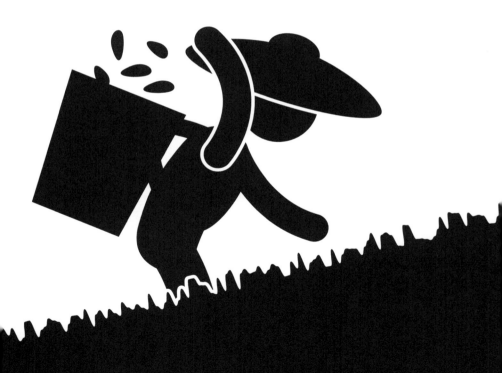

. . . i drink green tea over any other tea . . .

why?

the active ingredient in green tea, EGCG— a naturally occurring and potent antioxidant— increases the rate at which fat is burned in your body.

Green tea, which is one of the least processed teas, has many other benefits, including lowering cholesterol, but this antioxidant is key to weight loss.

Look for brands that contain sencha (ground green tea leaves); this means higher levels of the antioxidant EGCG. Most tea packaging has the level of antioxidant written on the box. I look for the highest levels when I am purchasing tea.

One to two cups of green tea have been proven to be beneficial to health. Five cups per day has been shown to boost weight loss, while 10 cups is my upper limit. Some is better than none—and I like the taste. It's also another source of hydration throughout the day.

Remember, most green teas contain caffeine, and, as with coffee, don't drink it if you suffer side effects.

rule #14

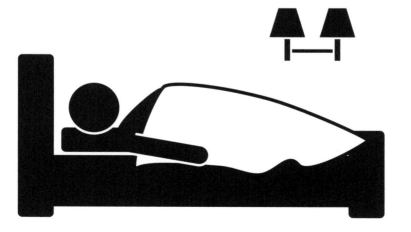

. . . i try to get nine hours of sleep a night . . .

sleep has been
shown to aid in
weight loss as
well as improving
your mental
well-being.

i like eight to nine
hours per night,
but try to aim for
seven and a half
hours at the
very least.

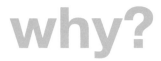

why?

we all need sleep— it's a no-brainer!

Eating and sleeping are two basic human functions, and they are closely intertwined. There are foods that promote sleep, such as leafy greens, and there are foods that inhibit sleep, such as fatty fast foods.

When I'm supertired, I make poor decisions for my weight, **like reaching for cookies or hunting through my daughter's bedroom to find the remnants of her party candy— desperate, really.**

It's self-sabotaging behavior, and I'm better off not exposing myself to it if I can help it. If I'm well rested, my brain is sharper and I have the willpower to keep going. When I first started my Big Weight Loss, I went to bed early, for two reasons. One, to stay away from food and break the bad habit of late-night eating, accu-

mulated over many years. Two, my research showed me the serious benefits of a good night's sleep. It helped that my nine-year-old liked that I was in bed early, too.

Personally, I like to sleep more in winter and find I require less sleep in summer. Our circadian rhythms can make us feel that way—so if you're sleeping more or less at different times of the year, don't worry about it. It's Mother Nature.

Sometimes, getting plenty of sleep simply isn't possible—I get that. Just do your best.

According to a study by scientists at Sweden's Uppsala University, lack of sleep can drastically slow your metabolism, causing weight gain. Yikes!

rule #15

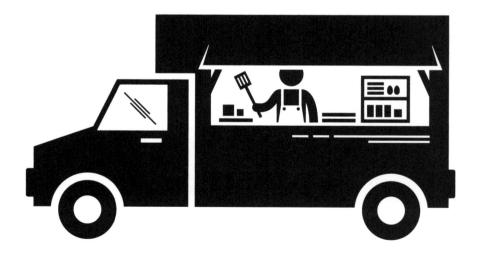

. . . I don't eat fast foods (usually) . . .

why?

Fast foods are cheap and convenient and, let's face it, can be damn tasty—when I'm actually eating them. But usually, after I've finished devouring them, I don't feel so great.

Unfortunately, fast food is filled mostly with sugar, bad fats and salt—not good for you. That's why you feel so terrible after you've eaten them, not to mention the guilt. Luckily, there are some exceptions . . . phew!

Such as:
Japanese: sushi, brown nori rolls
Vietnamese: low-carb rice paper rolls, pho
Lebanese: chicken or lamb and salad
Mexican: beans and salad and fish

Hunt around. There are plenty of good options once you know what to look for; think fresh, whole foods that are not deep fried.

you've gotta live in the real world! it's not possible to eat perfectly at every meal. sometimes you just need to eat something, quick.

just try to make smart choices when you're choosing what to put into your precious body. you're in control.

rule #16

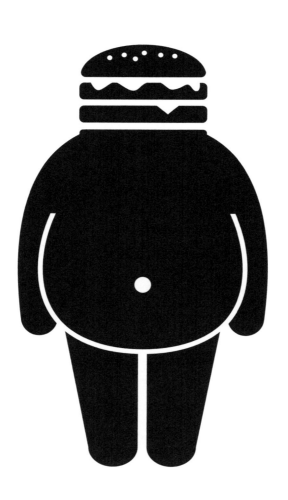

. . . i keep to a normal portion size . . .

food portion sizes have gone up and up over the past few decades.

before you go
back for more,
give yourself
twenty minutes
to digest what
you've eaten and
decide if you're
still hungry.

in other words,
wait. take a
breather—*you're
not going to
starve in the next
twenty minutes.*

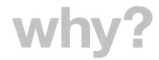

why?

The movie *Super Size Me* is a good example of out-of-control portions, particularly in fast foods. Not to mention the many other food-obsessed TV shows that celebrate the enormous portion sizes that have become almost commonplace in North America, Australia and the United Kingdom.

It's easy to control your portion sizes at home—but when eating out, it's tempting to consume everything you've been served, even after you've had enough. *Stop when you feel satisfied, not full*.

Remember, a piece of meat or fish should be the size of your palm, and the rest of the plate should be lots of veggies or salad. Follow it up with a piece of 80 percent dark chocolate or a small handful of nuts if you feel you need a little bit more.

It takes twenty minutes for the brain to get the signal from your stomach that you're full—that's a medical fact!

Try using a smaller plate; it will look like you've got a bigger portion. Plates have increased in size over the years, and the temptation is to fill the whole plate. Sounds dumb, but it actually works. Forget about set mealtimes; wait till you're actually hungry to eat—simple but effective.

rule #17

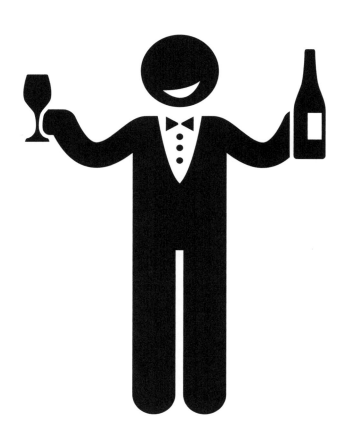

. . . i limit my alcohol . . .

why?

i'm not a big drinker, but occasionally i like to have a drink, and extra occasionally, i *really* like to have a drink — if you know what i mean.

I've ditched wine and champagne, which are both full of sugar that will convert and store straight to fat. Instead, I drink a vodka with lime soda, made with real limes and seltzer. Possibly on a night of dancing, I could get away with a bit more, as I would be burning up more energy.

I generally don't consume alcohol during the week. On the weekends, I may have one drink — but mostly it's easier to have none, as one can turn into three, which turns into six . . . And I'm more likely to eat unhealthy food if I'm drinking alcohol, so I try to avoid it.

And without alcohol, I wake up feeling fresher. This gets more and more true as I get older.

Admittedly, when I'm on vacation I loosen this rule . . . just a bit. What's a Bali sunset without a mojito with my friends? But try to avoid bad habits such as sinking a bottle of wine a night.

Alcohol also interferes with the way fat metabolizes — one more reason to limit it.

rule #18

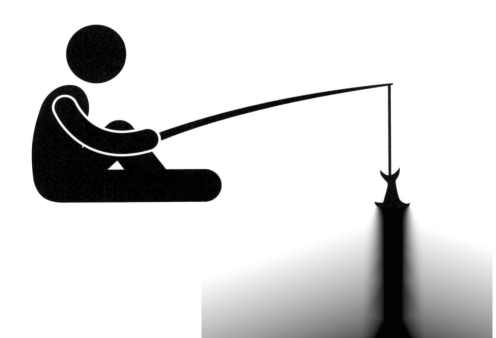

. . . i eat my leafy greens with a good fat . . . why?

eat your (large quantity of) leafy greens (seriously, go crazy on leafy greens) with a good fat such as avocado or a good-quality extra-virgin olive oil. this helps you absorb the vitamins. it's also tastier.

some examples of leafy greens are

Arugula

Kale

Lettuce

Spinach

Basically, if it's green and it's leafy, put it on your plate!

some examples of good natural fats are

Avocados

Salmon and oily fishes—sardines, etc.

Nuts

Natural nut butter (almond, peanut, etc.) with no salt or sugar added

Sunflower, sesame and pumpkin seeds

Olives

Extra-virgin olive oil

Cheese (in moderation)

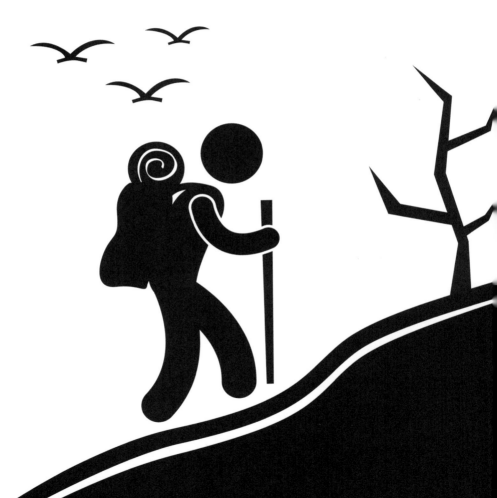

rule #19

. . . i always carry snacks . . .

when i'm out
or working on
location, i take
snacks with
me—i don't want
to get caught out
hungry with little
to choose from.

which?

Raw unprocessed nuts

Cut-up veggies

Berries

Hummus

Boiled eggs

Cheese

80 or 90 percent dark chocolate

Homemade smoothie: fresh fruit, veggies, ice/water

Raw unprocessed nuts—a healthy daily intake is 1 ounce or approximately ONE of the following serving sizes:

- 20 almonds
- 15 cashews
- 20 hazelnuts
- 15 macadamias
- 15 pecans
- 2 tablespoons of pine nuts
- 30 pistachio kernels
- 9 walnut kernels

A ziplock bag is my best friend, especially on fashion and advertising shoots. You should see the food that's offered: chocolate, candy, pastries . . . If I'm not prepared with my yummy snacks, then possible disaster.

rule #20

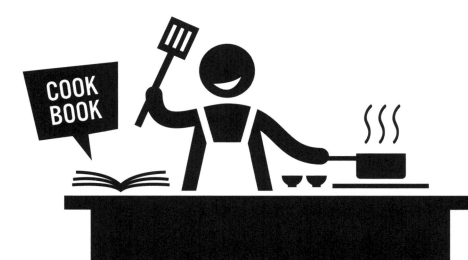

. . . prepare for your day/ week . . .

"by failing to prepare, you are preparing to fail."

—benjamin franklin

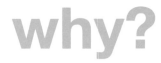

snacks

When you're out or at work and won't be able to access good food choices, bring snacks and lunch with you. I start eating at 10 a.m. every day, so I bring boiled eggs, nuts and two slices of Bern's Simple High-Protein Bread (page 33) with me.

shopping

It's easier to be healthy when you have all the right stuff in your cupboards and fridge. Keep your kitchen well stocked and junk free to make it easier to prepare meals for the whole family.

special occasions

When I'm going somewhere and I know there will be tempting foods, I try to eat beforehand. The hungrier I am, the less in control I am, to be honest. So I prevent that.

sweet

When I'm feeling in control, I will occasionally allow myself a small bit of something sweet. This can get out of control quickly, so I have to judge my mood and be honest with myself about how in control I really am. It's usually less than I think, in all honesty. Remember these two words: *special occasion*. This is not an everyday activity!

sometimes

Occasionally I double the amount of a meal I'm cooking and freeze half for another time—this is handy for times when I'm busy.

supermarkets

Don't go shopping hungry! It's a recipe for disaster.

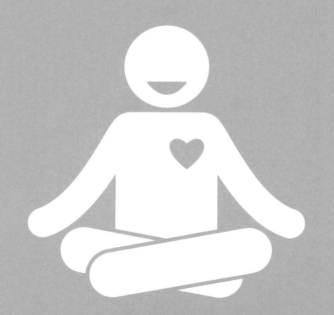

rules for the mind

sometimes i think that successful weight loss really starts in the mind.

rule #21

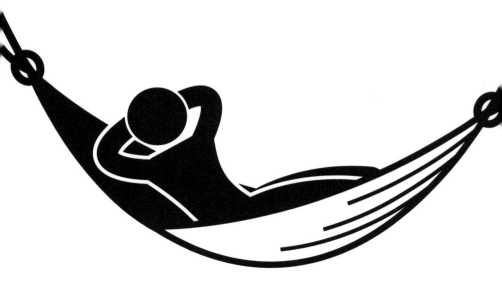

. . . i listen to my body . . .

why?

stop eating when you feel like you've had enough. remember, it takes twenty minutes for your brain to get the signal that you're full.

When you eat, focus on how your stomach feels through the entire meal. This is probably something that you will need to retrain yourself for, as you have probably been overeating for a while.

I had been overeating for, ooh, about twenty years. I remember I had to make a conscious effort to do this for the first couple of weeks of my Big Weight Loss.

As you become full, the empty feeling in your stomach will be replaced with a gentle pressure. As soon as you feel this, stop eating; if the fullness is uncomfortable, you overate.

And if you feel like throwing up or lying down, you really, really overate. It's all about listening to your body.

rule #22

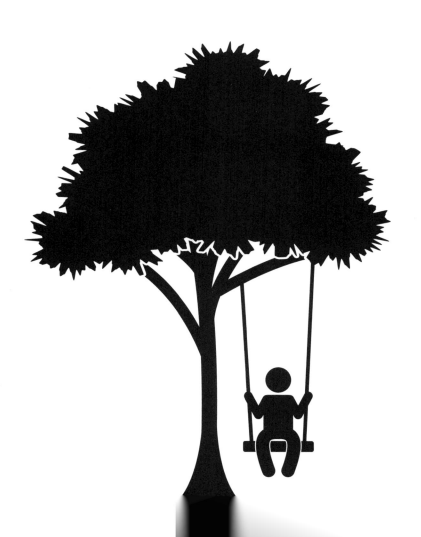

. . . I try my best not to get stressed . . .

stress makes you gain weight.

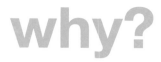

why?

it's all got to do with cortisol, a hormone released by your body in times of stress.

This reduces your anabolic hormones, in turn causing the body to store fat, slow your metabolic rate and increase your appetite. Nooooooooo!

This one's different for everybody, but for me, it's a definite weight gainer. When I was under considerable stress for a few years, I developed a tire around my upper stomach area.

Could it be that the stress made me want to eat more comfort foods? That was definitely true. But it's just as likely that the cortisol was kicking in and holding on to the fat.

Try to have fun and look at the lighter side of life. I also try to appreciate the little things, like the smells of spring, beautiful flowers, etc. I try to notice the good around me and take time out once in a while.

So don't stress the small stuff; it's not worth it.

rule #23

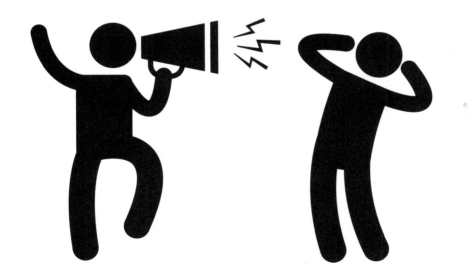

. . . i don't believe conventional wisdom about weight loss . . .

we can't believe
what we're told
about how to
lose weight when
there's an obesity
epidemic.

why?

make your own truth.

Conventional wisdom means those old sayings that you've heard a million times, like:

She's overweight, she must be lazy.
She doesn't have the willpower to lose weight.
Exercise more and eat less, and you'll lose weight.
Just exercise more.
Don't eat junk food.
Eat low fat.
Eat low calorie or count calories.
Eat six meals a day.
It's your fault you're fat.

These sayings are all flawed, and some are flat-out lies.

My personal favorite is "Eat low fat." That is crap! Most "low-fat" foods are filled with sugar and other nasties. Why on earth would you want to eat those? Unfortunately, we all bought into the "low-fat" diet fad.

Most of us consumed low-fat food believing that it must be better for us. This has turned out to be untrue, and the result has been a more obese society. Be your own guru. Actively pursue what works for you, using my rules as a starting point. Don't be swayed by extravagant weight loss claims that ask you to follow a crazy diet or buy expensive products. I've found that my own weight loss truth is actually pretty simple and surprisingly cheap—bonus!

rule #24

. . . hunger is not your friend . . .

it's not?

when you eat more
healthfully, you will
automatically feel full
for longer—healthy fats
and fiber help with that.

forget the old belief that
if you're feeling hungry,
you are somehow being
a good dieter.

it's not true.

It's emotionally taxing to fight hunger cravings, and you usually end up losing anyhow . . . then feel depressed . . . we've all been on that downward spiral.

Don't let yourself get too hungry or desperate for food. If you feel shaky, you've probably gone too long without eating—which ends up leading to poor decision making.

When you eat well, you should feel satisfied for about four hours. If you do get hungry, have a snack. Make sure you carry healthy nibbles with you at all times, just in case.

Know your weak times. For me, it's around 4 p.m., and sometimes, just after dinner. I make sure I'm prepared with 90 percent dark chocolate or some nuts.

It's harder to stick to a healthful, balanced diet when you're starving. It's much easier if you listen to your body and eat when you feel a bit hungry.

Give yourself every chance to succeed, and you will!

rule #25

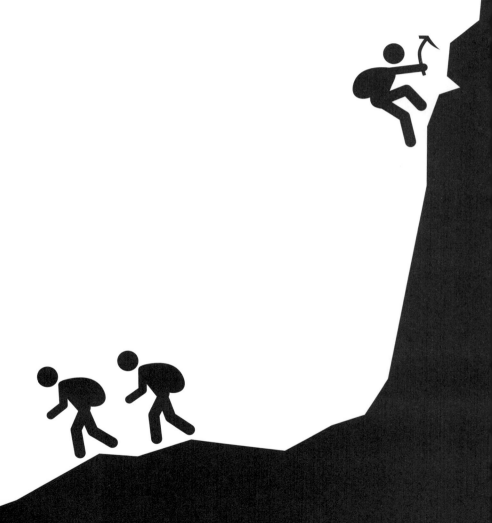

. . . i handle my sweet tooth cravings . . .

how?

once i stopped
consuming
truckloads of
sugar, my taste
buds adapted.
now i can taste
the real sweetness
in foods—even
vegetables.
isn't that amazing?

i no longer want extrasweet foods, as i find them too sweet. before i started the big weight loss, i was cynical of that claim—but it's true.

If you have a sweet tooth, then own it and be prepared. It's a good idea to make yourself a low-sugar treat such as melted 85 percent dark chocolate with nuts, coconut and seeds mixed in, then reset in the fridge. I always have something like this around. Sometimes I bake with fructose-free rice malt syrup or a little bit of unprocessed stevia. Other than these types of sweet snacks, don't torment yourself by keeping sugary stuff in the house—if it's available, it's easier to give in to temptation. Don't do that to yourself.

I recently went to a concert, and my partner bought me some normal chocolate to celebrate. (I know, WTF?) After eating a considerable amount (double WTF!) I nearly vomited. I felt really sick, really quickly. Lesson learned: I was NOT missing sugar. After that, it became even easier to say no to candy.

Look for dark chocolate with 80 to 90 percent cacao content. It contains minimal sugar (2.8 grams, or about half a teaspoon per serving), and because it has a strong taste, it's hard to pig out on.

Dark chocolate also has a host of health benefits (when eaten in moderation):

Cocoa beans contain flavonols, which have antioxidant effects that reduce the cell damage connected to heart disease, help lower blood pressure and improve vascular function.

There are more flavonols and less sugar in dark chocolate than milk chocolate. I eat two small pieces a day, as a treat.

rule #26

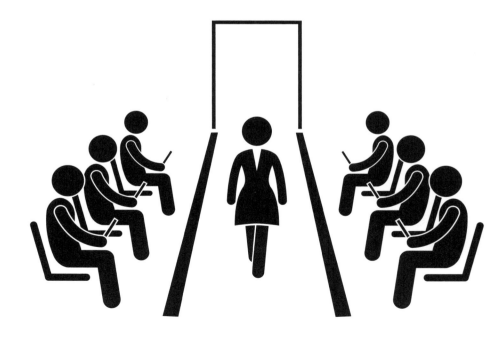

. . . don't aspire to unachievable media perfection . . .

hmmm?

it's hard to be
fat—in fact, it
really SUCKS.

how can you lose weight when supposedly healthful food is full of stuff that makes you fat? it's impossible.

As well as being unhealthy, there are so many social issues that go with being overweight. Most important, the majority of overweight people I know don't like their bodies at all and will constantly put themselves down. Women are experts at this.

It is so frustrating to lose weight and regain it, again and again. Then we blame ourselves for our failure. But by now you should know it's mostly not your fault—and I'm pretty pissed off at food companies. Cut yourself some slack—it's not all your doing.

There is such pressure, especially for young girls, to be beautiful and superslim like models in magazines. And I'm one of the people perpetuating that myth, as I do the hair and makeup that makes those models look the way they do. Before the picture is even taken, they usually spend at least one and a half hours in hair and makeup. Then the picture is Photoshopped for "flaws." What you see is absolutely not reality.

I remember working on an ad for a mainstream diet product overseas, and the model was gorgeous: tall, size 8 (US 4–6). The pictures were Photoshopped within an inch of her life because they thought her bum and legs looked too big—crazy! But it happens all the time.

To be perfectly honest, I'm not aiming for skinny. I much prefer the look of the models who are a healthy size 12–14 (US 10–12) with boobs and a bum—that's what I aspire to. Fit and curvy for me, please.

What I'm trying to say is, be the best that you can be—it's enough. In fact, it's more than enough.

rule #27

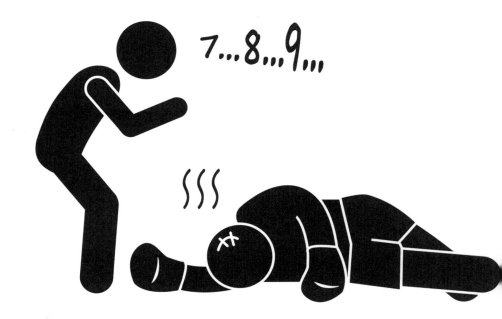

7...8...9...

. . . stop counting calories . . .

really?

it's annoying and time-consuming, and you don't need to when you eat according to my rules.

rule #28

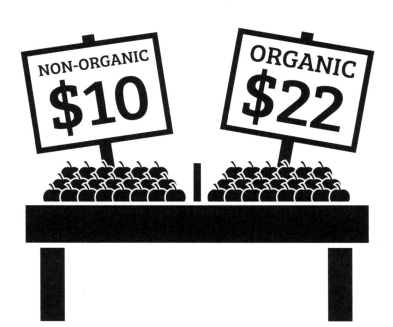

. . . organic is not necessarily better . . .

really?

organic whole foods are excellent—but processed organic foods are not.

Check the labels to make sure what you're eating is not high in hidden fats, sugars or chemicals.

Sometimes, the identical food is in the "normal" aisle at half the price—when ingredients are shelved in the health food area and stamped as organic, they suddenly cost double.

Some supposed health foods are really candy bars in disguise, with massive sugar content. Don't assume that the organic and health food aisle in the supermarket is all good— remember, read your food labels.

rule #29

. . . i use substitutes for white sugar . . . which?

I'm not crazy about artificial sweeteners; I find them too processed and the taste unpleasant. Here are some of them. Even the names of them sound unnatural. It's up to you, but I use them rarely.

- Saccharin
- Aspartame
- Acesulfame-K
- Sucralose
- Neotame

Plus, the jury is still out on whether artificial sweeteners are okay or harmful to your body in the long term. Why risk it?

The most natural artificial sweetener is stevia, which is a calorie-free plant extract 200 times as sweet as table sugar—a little goes a long way. Buy the least processed version of this possible. You can even grow it yourself.

I try to stay away from fructose in sugars (rule 1) and in general eat very little sugar. Sometimes, though, I really feel like something a bit sweet, and then I substitute either rice malt syrup, which is fructose free, or stevia instead of regular white sugar. Rice malt syrup is 100 percent glucose, which is still a form of sugar, and nutritionally it has few benefits other than being tasty, so I use it sparingly. Stevia is fructose free and is very low calorie, but sometimes I find it has a bit of an aftertaste. I use both of these substitutes only occasionally.

rule #30

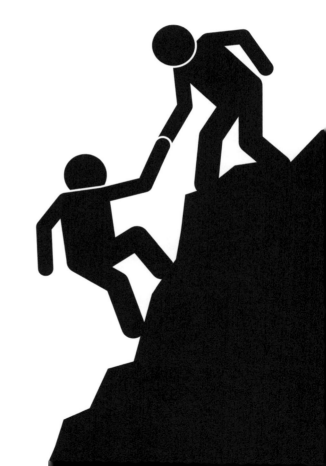

. . . be kind to yourself and think positively . . .

okay, then?

remember, if you slip up: tomorrow is another day and another chance to be healthy. in other words, be kind to yourself and *make yourself a priority.*

Go for a walk or take the kids on their scooters, just keep moving—it will help with your state of mind and make it easier to stay on track. Remember that *success is just outside of your comfort zone*—a total cliché but also totally true.

Sometimes I think that staying on track is more mental than anything else. If I'm angry or feeling flat or tired, it's easier to eat foods that are not good for me. **Yes, I'm a bit of an emotional eater.**

I believe that long-term weight loss is about changing your internal messages to yourself. Say to yourself: I can do it, you're doing well, good for you. Be your own best friend and coach; positive reinforcement will help you in the short and long term. *Positive actions lead to positive results.* Try to make this a daily habit.

I also find talking to other people about their healthy habits and sharing some of mine is inspiring. If you can find other people who are on the same healthy journey as you, even better. If you can surround yourself with positive people intent on positive change, that is fantastic. Talking helps—*we're all in this together!*

Visualize yourself living the life you want. *Believe you can do it—because you can.* Another totally true cliché!

rule #31

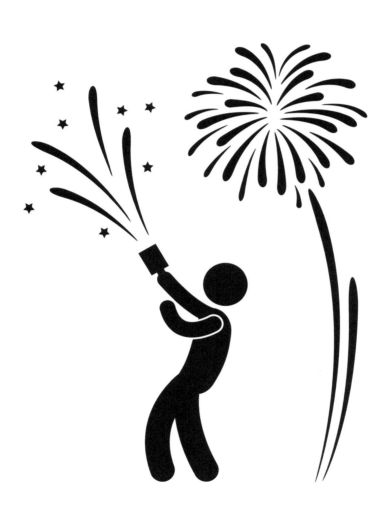

. . . celebrate your success and tolerate your plateaus . . .

why?

i reward myself with a
movie, clothes
or earrings—
anything but sugary
processed food. it's
almost enough of
a reward to see the
scales go down
and down.

It's about being good to yourself, being your own biggest champion. Do it because it's important—just as you are. I positively love shopping for clothes now. And I don't seem to be as invisible to shop assistants, for some reason. Funny!

While I'm transitioning between sizes, I buy my clothes at thrift stores or markets—I don't want to spend heaps on brand-new stuff I'm going to shrink out of. I also like eBay or factory outlets for this.

If your weight plateaus—i.e., you don't lose anything for a week—or three—don't worry. It's part of the weight loss journey and happens to everyone. I plateaued for more than three weeks, and, yes, it drove me crazy—but it did pass.

And after a weekend away hiking, I actually gained weight—3 pounds. Initially, I was super disappointed, as I had exercised and eaten well. But as my clothes were looser and I didn't feel as though I'd gained anything, I put it down to increased muscle (which weighs more than fat).

Sometimes the scales are wrong. Before you begin your Big Weight Loss journey, take your measurements and weight and put them into the "About You" section at the back of this book. Your shrinking measurements are another great way to see your progress.

how
to get
started

. . . take on one thing at a time . . .

. . . and take it one day at a time . . .

how to get started

Right before I first began this style of eating, I saw my doctor for blood tests and a check-up to see where I was at. After three months I saw her again, and we were both astounded at the improvements I had made.

It's a good idea to see your doctor before you start any weight loss plan—in case there is a medical issue you might not be aware of.

Next you'll need to do a big healthy shop at the market.

And you have to clean out your kitchen cupboards of all the unhealthy foods. Give them away, donate them, just get rid of them! If they're in the house, within arm's reach, it's far easier to give in to temptation.

Buy a pedometer, a smart watch or an app for your phone that counts steps. Devices that measure your sleep and steps are great. Get a good night's sleep, then get up and weigh and measure yourself—you're good to go with the first step.

Week by week, I took on one hard task and one easy task, until I was doing all these habits together. This achieved the fastest weight loss possible. Obviously it's going to vary from person to person, depending on your habits and what you find hard and easy.

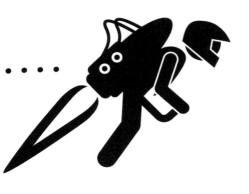

week 1

I started off by getting rid of processed foods and adding what I thought was an easy habit: walking.

week 2

I gave up sugar (a harder one for me) and added in good sleeping habits.

week 3

I cut back on my carbs and added another easy one: no soda.

And so on. Introducing new things each week gives you the best chance of success. Some weeks are going to be easier than others—expect that, but persevere. The payoff will be weight loss—lots of it.

However you approach this, you're off and running to a healthier and slimmer you.

perseverance and persistence are key.

what's in my cupboards and fridge

dairy products

Eggs—free range

Yogurt (full-fat Greek)

Milk (full fat)

Sour cream

Cheese—I love soft feta and haloumi

Butter/ghee

vegetables

Cauliflower (good for cauliflower rice)

Avocado

Carrots

Red peppers—I roast these

Sweet potatoes

Zucchini—for spiralizing

Tomatoes—I like cherry ones

Pumpkin—love it roasted

Leafy greens—lots of them

Mushrooms—yum on toast at breakfast

Whatever else you like—I do not tend to buy corn or white potatoes

fruit

Berries

Apples

Oranges

Seasonal fruits

meat and fish

Pork (free range and organic)

Beef (grass fed)

Salmon and fresh white fish—if I have the $!

Tuna (canned, ethically caught)

Chicken (organic)

Bacon (free range and organic)

nuts, legumes and seeds

Nuts—buy a variety of raw and unsalted ones

Lentils—a variety of dried and canned

Beans—a variety of dried and canned

Pumpkin seeds—I use these in baking bread

liquids

Coconut oil (raw and organic)

Olive oil

Rice malt syrup

Balsamic vinegar

Coconut milk and cream

Apple cider vinegar with mother

Stevia—the most natural and unprocessed

pantry

Flours—lentil, chickpea, coconut

Chia seeds, quinoa

Rice (brown or wild)

Oats (rolled, plain and unsweetened)

Herbs and spices

Nut butters like almond or peanut butter with no added sugars or salt

Dark chocolate with 80–90 percent cacao

Green tea bags

Coffee

Bottles of seltzer

Small ziplock bags

an example of a typical day, foodwise

drink water first thing, with all meals and throughout the day, as well as green tea.

7 a.m.—first thing

Coffee with a dash of full-fat milk or coconut milk (sometimes I have two)

10 a.m.—breakfast—this is when i first eat

One of the following:
- 2 pieces protein or whole grain bread, ½ avocado, 2 slices bacon
- 1 piece protein or whole grain bread, 2 poached eggs
- 1 ounce rolled oats with yogurt and berries
- 1 tablespoon chia seeds with yoghurt and berries
- 2 pieces protein or whole grain bread, grilled with cheese and tomato
- 2 eggs scrambled in butter, mushrooms, spinach
- Steamed green veggies with soft feta and nuts

2 p.m.—lunch—it's quite simply a mix of protein and leafy greens (think ¼ protein and ¾ leafy greens)

One of the following:
- A large bowl of soup—homemade with veggies or beans
- A large green salad with salmon or chicken
- Any combo of leafy greens and a palm-size portion of protein
- Salmon sashimi—I love Japanese food

4 p.m.—snack

One of the following:
- 1 ounce nuts—raw and unsalted
- Berries—a small handful

6 p.m.—dinner

One of the following:
- Grilled fish or meat with vegetables or salad
- Coconut milk Thai curry—made with fish, chicken or vegetables and served with cauliflower rice
- Indian curry—as above
- Leafy greens with onion, tomato and fresh Parmesan, dressed with olive oil and balsamic vinegar

6:45 p.m.—snack

2 pieces of 85 percent dark chocolate

No eating after 7 p.m.

If you find it difficult to stick to these times, have your breakfast as late as possible and your dinner as early as possible. I also don't see anything wrong with skipping breakfast if you have had a late dinner the night before. Remember, just do your best!

finally . . .

you don't
need luck,
this will
work

don't go back to your previous bad habits and bad eating. learn what feels good for your body and mind and stick to it, because you deserve it.

Lots of people lose weight on fad diets, only to regain it within five years—and more. Look at *The Biggest Loser* statistics—many of the contestants have regained the weight they lost, because in the real world it's not possible to exercise for hours each day. Who has that much free time? No one! My life is generally messy and busy.

Weight loss needs to be achievable. It's a long-term lifestyle change. Don't be one of those statistics—you will need to consistently stay away from sugar and processed foods.

It's a fine balance; if I'm feeling the desire to eat sugary foods, I know I need to wipe everything sweet off the menu for a bit. Sugar is seriously addictive for me.

Twice a week, I weigh myself in my bra and underwear so that I can keep an eye on my progress. If I can do this, so can you.

believe in yourself.

maintenance

Once you've hit your goal weight or size, you can think about adding back a little bit more fruit, or a few more carbs—or maybe don't do the intermittent fast every night. It's really up to you.

You're going to give your body more of the healthful and nutritious foods that it deserves. I believe you won't fall back into bad habits because you will have learned what feels good for your body. And you're on a lifelong path to good health.

Find a balance in food and lifestyle that you can live with for life. The best possible life. Good luck!

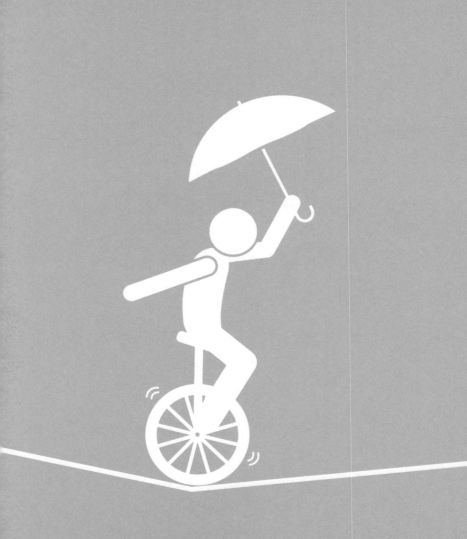

just some of the many medical studies i've read

Acheson, K. J., B. Zahorska-Markiewicz, P. Pittet, K. Anantharaman, and E. Jéquier. "Caffeine and Coffee: Their Influence on Metabolic Rate and Substrate Utilization in Normal Weight and Obese Individuals." *The American Journal of Clinical Nutrition* 33, no. 5 (May 1980): 989–97.

Avena, Nicole M., Pedro Rada, and Bartley G. Hoebel. "Evidence for Sugar Addiction: Behavioral and Neurochemical Effects of Intermittent, Excessive Sugar Intake." *Neuroscience and Biobehavioral Reviews* 32, no. 1 (2008): 20–39. doi: 10.1016/j.neubiorev.2007.04.019.

Benedict, Christian, Manfred Hallschmid, Arne Lassen, et al. "Acute Sleep Deprivation Reduces Energy Expenditure in Healthy Men." *The American Journal of Clinical Nutrition* 93, no. 6 (April 6, 2011): 1229–36. doi: 10.3945/ajcn.110.006460.

Cawley, John, and Chad Meyerhoefer. "The Medical Care Costs of Obesity: An Instrumental Variables Approach." *Journal of Health Economics* 31, no. 1 (2012): 219–30.

DiNicolantonio, James J., and Sean C. Lucan. "The Wrong White Crystals: Not Salt but Sugar as Aetiological in Hypertension and Cardiometabolic Disease." *Open Heart* 1 (2014); 1:e000167. doi: 10.1136/openhrt-2014–000167.

Finkelstein, Eric A., Justin G. Trogdon, Joel W. Cohen, and William Dietz. "Annual Medical Spending Attributable to Obesity: Payer—and Service-Specific Estimates." *Health Affairs* 36, no. 6 (2009): 822–31.

Glickman, Dan, Lynn Parker, Leslie J. Sim, Heather Del Valle Cook, and Emily Ann Miller, eds. *Accelerating Progress in Obesity Prevention: Solving the Weight of the Nation*. Washington, DC: National Academies Press, 2012.

Hankey, Catherine, Dominika Klukowska, and Michael Lean. "A Systematic Review of the Literature on Intermittent Fasting for Weight Management." *The FASEB Journal* 29, no. 1 (suppl.) (April 2015): 117.4.

Howarth, Nancy C., Edward Saltzman, and Susan B. Roberts. "Dietary Fiber and Weight Regulation." *Nutrition Reviews* 59, no. 5 (May 2001): 129–39. doi: 10.1111/j.1753-4887.2001.tb07001.x.

Hung, Hsin-Chia., et al., "Fruit and Vegetable Intake and Risk of Major Chronic Disease." *Journal of the National Cancer Institute* 96, no. 21 (2004): 1577–84.

Jacobson, Michael F. "Liquid Candy: How Soft Drinks Are Harming Americans' Health." Washington, DC: Center for Science in the Public Interest, 2005.

Ludwig, David S., Karen E. Peterson, and Steven L. Gortmaker. "Relation Between Consumption of Sugar-Sweetened Drinks and Childhood Obesity: A Prospective, Observational Analysis." *The Lancet* 357 (February 17, 2001): 505–8. doi: http://dx.doi.org/10.1016/S0140–6736(00)04041–1.

Mozaffarian, Dariush, Tao Hao, Eric B. Rimm, and Frank B. Wu. "Changes in Diet and Lifestyle and Long-term Weight Gain in Women and Men." *New England Journal of Medicine* 364 (June 2011): 2392–2404. doi: 10.1056/NEJMoa1014296.

Patel, Sanjay R., Atul Malhotra, David P. White, Daniel J. Gottlieb, and Frank B. Hu. "Association Between Reduced Sleep and Weight Gain in Women." *American Journal of Epidemiology* 164, no. 10 (November 15, 2006): 947–54.

Stookey, Jodi D., Florence Constant, Barry M. Popkin, and Christopher D. Gardner. "Drinking Water Is Associated with Weight Loss in Overweight Dieting Women Independent of Diet and Activity." *Obesity* 16 (September 2008): 2481–88. doi: 10.1038/oby.2008.409.

University of Minnesota. "15-year Study Shows Strong Link Between Fast Food, Obesity and Insulin Resistance." ScienceDaily, 19 January 2005. www.sciencedaily.com/releases/2005/01/050111152135.htm.

Venables, Michael C., Carl J. Hulston, Hannah R. Cox, and Asker E. Jeukendrup. "Green Tea Extract Ingestion, Fat Oxidation, and Glucose Tolerance in Healthy Humans." *The American Journal of Clinical Nutrition* 87 (March 2008): 778–84.

Wansink, Brian, and Koert van Ittersum. "The Visual Illusions of Food: Why Plates, Bowls, and Spoons Can Bias Consumption Volume." *FASE Journal* 20 (Meeting Abstract Supplement) A618 (March 2006).

World Cancer Research Fund/American Institute for Cancer Research. *Food, Nutrition, Physical Activity, and the Prevention of Cancer: A Global Perspective*. Washington, DC: American Institute for Cancer Research, 2007.

thanks to

Terence Langendoen, Lilli Langendoen, Claire Fisers, Jakki and Johann Bilsborough, Myrtle Jeffs, Mel Krienke, Claryssa Humennyj-Jameson, Kylie Starling, Felicite Phillips, Michael Heath, Harriet Reuter Hapgood, Christian Lockwood, Jack Lockwood, Michael Lenihan, Julie Spalding, Lisa Tyler, Natalie Kirby, Susan Whitlam, Virginya Thomas, Zoe King, Olivia Maidment, Amy Fitzgerald, Mirette Al Rafie, Georgie Mellor plus everyone at The Blair Partnership London, all my publishers and publicists worldwide including Megan Beatie, Cara Bedick, Lara Blackman, Sydney Morris, Susan Moldow, David Falk, Tara Parsons, and all the Touchstone US staff, plus all the models, art directors, clients, athletes, trainers and photographers I have worked with who have talked to me about nutrition and have encouraged me—I thank you all.

follow bernadette online

 @bigweightlossau

 @littlebookbigweightloss

 @littlebookofbigweightloss

 pinterest.com/bernfish/the-little-book-of-big-weightloss/